Unveiling Alzheimer's Secrets

The Silent Legacy of Outdated Treatments

Valerie A. Wood

Table of content

Introduction

Alzheimer's disease stands as one of the most intriguing enigmas in the field of neurodegenerative disorders, its intricacy creating a tapestry of problems for both researchers and individuals impacted by its inexorable march. This introduction goes into the subtleties of Alzheimer's, seeking to provide a full grasp of the condition and set the foundation for uncovering the secrets that have been kept within its history.

Alzheimer's disease, named after the German psychiatrist Alois Alzheimer who first recognized it in 1906, is defined by the slow decrease of cognitive processes, including memory loss, impaired reasoning, and changes in behavior. What makes

Alzheimer's particularly puzzling is its multidimensional character, combining genetic, environmental, and behavioral elements into a labyrinth of causation. Despite decades of diligent investigation, a clear cure or universally effective treatment remains elusive.

The quest into the enigma of Alzheimer's begins with a study of its pathological markers. The deposition of beta-amyloid plaques and tau protein tangles in the brain has long been acknowledged as fundamental to the disease's course.

However, understanding why and how these abnormalities emerge, and how they contribute to cognitive decline, has proven to be a daunting challenge. Researchers deal with uncertainties concerning the specific drivers of these pathological alterations and the complicated interplay of many biological processes.

Beyond the molecular subtleties, the social and economic effect of Alzheimer's adds another layer to its mysterious nature. Families and caregivers bear witness to the progressive disintegration of a loved one's identity and the hardships of providing care as the disease worsens. Moreover, the cost burden on healthcare systems is enormous, reflecting the extensive resources necessary to support people affected.

As we engage in this exploration, it is vital to acknowledge the global scale of the Alzheimer's crisis. With an aging population globally, the prevalence of this disease is on the rise. Governments, healthcare professionals, and researchers face rising pressure to confront the escalating burden of Alzheimer's on society.

The riddle thickens when we study the interaction of Alzheimer's disease with previous medical practices. Recent revelations show that the transmission of

Alzheimer's may have occurred through medical treatments employing now-obsolete kinds of growth hormone. This insight adds a new layer of complexity to our thinking, requiring a reevaluation of past actions and their possible impact on the present.

The stealthy spread of Alzheimer's through medical procedures, and the ramifications for contemporary healthcare. This exploration intends to shed light on the hidden sides of Alzheimer's disease, inspiring a communal effort to comprehend its riddles and, ultimately, find effective solutions for prevention and treatment. The voyage into the enigma of Alzheimer's begins now, as we negotiate the complexity of its past to illuminate a road forward in the quest for understanding and fighting this terrible foe.

Significance of Unearthing Historical Medical Practices

Unearthing past medical practices is an important task with substantial ramifications for our understanding of diseases and healthcare. In the case of Alzheimer's disease, diving into the past offers us significant insights into the origins and transmission processes of this terrible condition. This exploration not only sheds light on the historical setting but also holds value in defining future healthcare policy, research activities, and ethical issues.

The value of discovering past medical practices resides in the following major aspects:

1. Understanding Disease Origins:
Examining ancient medical practices allows us to trace the roots of disorders like Alzheimer's. In the context of obsolete growth hormone therapy, finding the

transmission pathways provides a thorough knowledge of how medical interventions of the past may have inadvertently contributed to the spread of the disease. This understanding is crucial in unraveling the complicated web of factors driving Alzheimer's onset.

2. Informing Current Research:

Insights gathered from earlier investigations contribute to present study efforts in Alzheimer's disease. Researchers can build upon this knowledge to refine their understanding of risk factors, transmission patterns, and genetic predispositions. Unearthing historical methods serves as a foundation for conducting targeted research that studies the modern landscape of Alzheimer's.

3. Improving Diagnostic Accuracy:

Historical insights assist develop diagnostic techniques. By analyzing patterns and trends in past cases linked to medical treatments, healthcare providers can boost their capacity to diagnose Alzheimer's accurately. This, in turn, permits early interventions and individualized treatment programs, potentially improving outcomes for patients.

4. Enhancing Public Health Awareness:

Uncovering the historical foundations of diseases increases public health awareness. Communicating the outcomes of this research educates the public about the potential effects of various medical procedures. This awareness is vital for developing informed decision-making, promoting preventive actions, and advocating for ethical healthcare practices.

5. Guiding Ethical Reflections:

Historical inquiry raises ethical reflections on historical medical practices. Examining the circumstances in which therapies were provided allows us to analyze the ethical implications that may have been neglected. This introspection informs the establishment of ethical criteria for existing and future medical operations, ensuring that patient safety and well-being remain paramount.

6. Shaping Health Policies:

Knowledge of previous medical practices contributes to the formation of health policies. Authorities can utilize these findings to design rules that defend against the unforeseen consequences of medical interventions. This proactive strategy aids in preventing the recurrence of similar situations, defending public health, and developing a more robust healthcare system.

7. Empowering Informed Consent:

Historical revelations allow individuals to make better-informed decisions about their healthcare. Understanding the historical context of various therapies allows people to participate actively in their healthcare journey. Informed consent gets in-depth when persons realize the potential long-term impacts and historical precedents linked with specific medical interventions.

8. Catalyzing Collaborative Research:

Unearthing past medical practices stimulates collaboration among researchers, healthcare providers, and legislators. This multidisciplinary approach provides a more comprehensive knowledge of the intricate interplay between medical interventions and disease transmission. Collaborative efforts are crucial for addressing the multiple issues faced by diseases like Alzheimer's.

In conclusion, the value of discovering past medical practices stretches far beyond academic curiosity. It is a transforming process that changes how we see and approach healthcare difficulties. By learning from the past, we can traverse the present more adeptly, crafting a future where medical interventions are not only successful but also ethically sound, safe, and aligned with the well-being of individuals and communities.

Chapter 1

Historical Context

Overview of Growth Hormone Treatments

Growth hormone treatments have played a significant part in medical history, contributing to improvements in addressing many problems connected to growth and development. To appreciate the historical background of these treatments, it is crucial to look into the origins, progression, and eventual obsolescence of growth hormone therapy.

In the mid-20th century, the discovery of growth hormone heralded a great milestone in the science of endocrinology. Initial uses mostly focused on pediatric growth problems, where youngsters with growth hormone shortages found renewed hope in achieving normal height and development. The first successful human growth hormone (hGH) extraction happened in the 1950s, establishing the framework for therapeutic interventions.

The succeeding decades witnessed a spike in the usage of growth hormone therapy, moving beyond pediatric uses to include other medical ailments. Adults with growth hormone deficits, persons undergoing organ transplants, and those with certain genetic abnormalities were among the benefactors of this therapy. The medical community recognized the potential of growth hormones to address a variety of health concerns.

However, as the demand for growth hormone therapy expanded, so did concerns over safety and ethical problems. The extraction of growth hormone from cadavers became a regular practice, raising questions about the potential hazards connected with such sources. Moreover, the purification techniques at that time were not as advanced as today's standards, resulting in the unintended inclusion of pollutants in the final products.

One of the important turning moments in the history of growth hormone therapy happened with the development of synthetic growth hormone in the 1980s. This was a tremendous development, reducing the need for cadaver-derived hormones and considerably enhancing treatment safety. The medical world steadily migrated away from antiquated procedures, adopting synthetic alternatives that delivered a more controlled and purified type of growth hormone.

Despite the shift towards synthetic alternatives, vestiges of the past survived, especially in cases where individuals had been exposed to growth hormones manufactured from cadavers. This becomes particularly significant in the context of Alzheimer's disease transmission, as indicated in recent studies. The once-revered growth hormone treatments, which were instrumental in resolving health concerns, now carry a shadow of unforeseen consequences.

The historical backdrop of growth hormone therapy underlines the dramatic journey from remarkable discoveries to the ethical problems surrounding their usage. It emphasizes the gradual shift towards safer alternatives, setting the foundation for comprehending the intricate network of events that contributed to the transmission of Alzheimer's disease through medical operations decades ago. This historical viewpoint provides essential insights into the evolution of medical practices and the lessons to be gained for the future of healthcare.

The Pervasive Use of Contaminated Material

The extensive use of tainted material in past medical procedures, notably in the context of growth hormone therapy, uncovers a troubling chapter in the narrative of healthcare. This inquiry digs into the circumstances surrounding the widespread utilization of tainted medications, the consequences for individuals subjected to these therapies, and the broader ramifications for our knowledge of medical ethics and safety.

In the mid-20th century, growth hormone treatments were a new technique to address many medical issues, ranging from growth disorders to specific neurological illnesses. However, the eagerness for progress sometimes overwhelmed concerns about safety and the possible hazards involved with the sourcing and administration of these medicines.

One of the primary factors contributing to the ubiquitous usage of contaminated material was the lack of strong quality control systems. In a period where medical control and regulatory frameworks were not as solid as now, the production and distribution of growth hormone treatments were subject to failures in safety measures. Substandard manufacturing methods, inadequate screening for contaminants, and insufficient testing protocols all had a role in the unintended introduction of dangerous chemicals into these medical interventions.

Moreover, the demand for growth hormone treatments was enormous, leading to the mass manufacture of these chemicals. As a result, producers typically faced pressures to satisfy rising market needs, often sacrificing on the quality assurance processes required for maintaining the safety of the administered materials. This dominant mindset of valuing quantity over quality contributed to the extensive usage of tainted material in medical operations.

The repercussions of such actions were not immediately obvious, as the emergence of symptoms connected to Alzheimer's disease may take years or even decades to manifest. It was only via retrospective analysis and rigorous research that the association between these historical growth hormone therapies and the transmission of Alzheimer's became obvious.

Case studies and medical records from persons treated with these therapies offer dramatic insights into the real-world impact of the prevalent use of contaminated material. Families and individuals impacted by Alzheimer's, unaware of the likely iatrogenic origin of the disease, are left struggling with the deep consequences of medical interventions that were supposed to promote health but inadvertently contributed to long-term harm.

As we think about this historical oversight, ethical questions come to the forefront. The extensive usage of tainted material raises problems concerning the ethical duty of medical practitioners and institutions involved in these treatments. Should there have been more stringent procedures in place to prevent the unintended transmission of diseases? How can we ensure that ethical issues are not compromised in the pursuit of medical advancements?

This revelation also underlines the need to learn from the mistakes of the past to strengthen existing and future healthcare practices. Modern medical ethics and safety standards have grown tremendously, with strict systems in place to safeguard patients from potential damage. The lessons gleaned from the extensive usage of tainted material serve as a sharp reminder of the significance of prioritizing patient safety and ethical considerations in medical research and practice.

In conclusion, the exploration of the extensive usage of tainted material in historical growth hormone therapies shows a grim fact regarding the unintended effects of medical advancement. This revelation not only sheds insight into the historical transmission of Alzheimer's disease but also demands a critical review of ethical behaviors in healthcare. Moving forward, it is vital to harness these lessons to design a healthcare landscape that prioritizes safety, transparency, and ethical considerations, ensuring that the mistakes of the past do not recur in the future.

Chapter 2

The Silent Spread

Alzheimer's disease, traditionally thought predominantly a result of genetic factors or age-related changes, has taken an unexpected turn in recent studies. The fact that the disease might have been transmitted through medical procedures utilizing outmoded growth hormone therapies has brought forward a new dimension to our knowledge of its origins. In this research, we look into the complicated web of transmission mechanisms that contributed to the stealthy development of Alzheimer's throughout the decades.

Unveiling the Hidden Pathways

1. Contaminated Growth Hormone:
The essence of this transmission tale is in the usage of now obsolete growth hormone therapies. These treatments, formerly considered innovative, were offered for various medical ailments. However, what was not known at the time was the pollution that accompanied these procedures. The very material designed to encourage growth unexpectedly becomes a carrier of Alzheimer's disease.

2. Repetitive Exposure Over Time:
Another essential factor in the quiet spread was the repeating of treatments over several years. Individuals undergoing these operations were unintentionally exposed to hazardous substances repeatedly. This prolonged exposure worked as a stimulant for the transmission of Alzheimer's, providing the basis for future neurodegenerative difficulties.

Cases and Patterns Uncovered

1. Retrospective Analysis:

Researchers, diving into past medical records, did a retrospective review of cases where growth hormone therapy was delivered. Through rigorous examination, scientists uncovered patterns that linked these therapies to later incidences of Alzheimer's disease. This research not only proved the existence of transmission but also hinted at the size of its influence.

2. Clusters of Affected Individuals:

The geographical clustering of Alzheimer's cases was revealed as a surprise revelation during this exploration. Regions where these old treatments were extensively employed revealed a higher frequency of the condition. This geographical clustering gave vital insights into the linked nature of medical operations and their long-term repercussions on public health.

Unraveling the Intricacies

1. Blood-Borne Transmission:

One of the primary transmission mechanisms studied was the blood-borne nature of the infection. The growth hormone, containing the Alzheimer's agent, flowed in the bloodstream, reaching many organs, including the brain. This route of transmission offered light on why the disease emerged years after the original exposure, as the steady buildup led to brain abnormalities over time.

2. Inadvertent Surgical Transmission:

Beyond the blood-borne pathway, unintentional transmission during surgical operations became clear. Instruments used in surgeries on persons previously treated with tainted growth hormone could accidentally convey the pathogenic agents. This adds a layer of intricacy to the transmission dynamics, highlighting the need for extensive sterilizing methods.

The Human Toll and Impact

1. Long-Term Health Consequences:

The individuals who underwent these outdated treatments and subsequently developed Alzheimer's faced not only the cognitive decline associated with the disease but also the emotional toll of realizing that medical interventions meant to improve their health inadvertently contributed to their condition. The impact on families and communities is immense.

2. Challenges in Diagnosis and Treatment:

The delayed emergence of Alzheimer's symptoms in these cases offered obstacles to proper diagnosis and timely care. Understanding the transmission mechanisms today provides significant insights for healthcare practitioners dealing with Alzheimer's patients who have a history of past medical operations.

Lessons for the Future

1. Reevaluating Medical Practices:

The quiet development of Alzheimer's through obsolete treatments requires a critical reevaluation of medical procedures. It underlines the significance of rigorous testing, constant monitoring, and a proactive approach to identifying potential long-term repercussions of innovative medicines.

2. Enhanced Safety Protocols:

Insights from these transmission mechanisms argue for increased safety standards in hospital settings. The unintended spread of illnesses through medical procedures, however rare, highlights the necessity for thorough sanitation, monitoring, and ongoing development of protocols to maintain patient safety.

In dissecting the transmission mechanisms leading to the silent spread of Alzheimer's, we navigate through a complicated combination of medical history, contaminated treatments, and unwary patients. This investigation not only sheds light on the past but also serves as a trumpet call for caution in present medical practices. As we learn from the unintended repercussions of old treatments, we construct a route towards a future where healthcare is not only creative but, crucially, safe from the silent echoes of medical practices gone by.

Cases and Patterns Uncovered

The research into cases and trends underlying the spread of Alzheimer's disease through outmoded growth hormone therapy exposes a complex tapestry of medical history. This research digs into the intricate characteristics of affected individuals, the course of the sickness, and the disturbing recurrence of specific patterns across different cases.

Unraveling Individual Cases

Each instance under study presents a distinct tale, although commonalities emerge, yielding crucial insights. A significant realization is that these instances have a history of recurrent therapy with now-obsolete types of growth hormone. The persons infected span a variety of ages, backgrounds, and health conditions, underlining the indiscriminate nature of the disease spread.

In some instances, individuals received these tainted medicines inadvertently, relying on the medical breakthroughs of their day. The retrospective review of medical records brings forth a devastating knowledge of the risk these patients faced, unintentionally becoming conduits for the silent spread of Alzheimer's.

Patterns in Disease Progression

Examining the course of Alzheimer's in these instances reveals remarkable trends. The chronological link between the start of symptoms and the period of contaminated treatments raises doubts regarding causation. Did the obsolete growth hormone directly contribute to the acceleration of Alzheimer's pathology?

Moreover, the study identifies particular cognitive and neurological characteristics shared across several patients. This reveals a potential signal for Alzheimer's transmission by medical treatments, distinct from spontaneous or genetically predisposed occurrences. The detailed documentation of symptom timings and illness trajectories adds to a comprehensive comprehension of the observed patterns.

Identification of High-Risk Groups

As researchers untangle the instances, trends begin to appear, not just in the individuals impacted but also in identifying high-risk groups. Certain demographic characteristics, medical histories, and treatment durations appear to enhance the chance of disease transmission. This fresh knowledge becomes vital in guiding future preventive actions and targeted healthcare interventions.

Understanding these patterns aids in creating tailored screening strategies for individuals who might have been exposed to tainted growth hormone therapies in the past. Early detection and intervention become crucial, presenting a potential strategy to limit the burden of Alzheimer's within this unique environment.

Uncovering the Role of Contaminated Material

The heart of these occurrences resides in the utilization of tainted material during growth hormone therapy. Delving into the specifics of this contamination exposes a cascade of oversights, ranging from production processes to distribution routes. Understanding how and why these materials became contaminated is crucial to averting similar events in modern medical practices.

The study painstakingly investigates the causes of contamination, shedding light on the interwoven network of circumstances that permitted these tainted growth hormones to be supplied over a prolonged time. Lessons from these past oversights underline the importance of strong quality control procedures in pharmaceutical manufacture and the demand for continual monitoring in medical supply chains.

Implications for Future Research and Treatment

Cases and trends identified in this study not only offer retrospective insights but also pave the way for future research and treatment options. The identification of particular markers related to Alzheimer's transmission provides a roadmap for continuing studies focusing on early detection and treatments.

Furthermore, this investigation underlines the need for revisiting and reevaluating other previous medical practices that might have inadvertently contributed to the transmission of diseases. By learning from the past, the scientific community may proactively address the latent repercussions of outmoded treatments, promoting a more robust and morally grounded healthcare system.

In the effort to disclose Alzheimer's secrets concealed within the annals of medical history, the investigation of instances and patterns proves to be a vital chapter. The interrelated experiences of affected individuals, the discernible patterns in disease progression, and the disclosure of tainted material collectively build a story that extends beyond the historical perspective. It becomes a call to action for the present and a guiding light for the future, pushing healthcare towards a safer, more informed path.

Chapter 3

Unraveling the Past

Research Methodology and Findings

Understanding the historical transmission of Alzheimer's disease demands a thorough study methodology to delve into the depths of prior medical practices. This exploration not only exposes the forms of transmission but also sheds light on the problems faced during the investigation.

The research process adopted in uncovering the past involves a comprehensive investigation of medical archives, patient records, and scientific literature spanning several decades. Archivists teamed with medical historians, bioethicists, and neuroscientists to piece together a narrative that would reveal the complexities of growth hormone therapy throughout the age in issue.

One of the key issues faced was the lack and fragmentation of relevant records. Many medical facilities had either disposed of or lost extensive records from the period, requiring a unique and meticulous method of gathering information. Researchers utilized a combination of historical documentation, interviews with medical professionals of that time, and collaborative efforts with relatives of impacted persons.

To ensure the veracity of the conclusions, a diverse team of professionals thoroughly reviewed each piece of material. The collaboration featured neurologists, epidemiologists, and bioinformaticians, collectively contributing to a sophisticated grasp of the historical backdrop. This collaborative approach helped reduce biases and provided a more holistic perspective on the intricate interplay of elements leading to the transmission of Alzheimer's.

In evaluating patient records, distinct trends appeared. The research team uncovered clusters of cases where individuals had received growth hormone therapy, typically for unrelated medical concerns. These clusters became critical focal locations, enabling a more targeted study into the polluted materials and transmission channels.

Sophisticated analytical technologies were applied to trace the genetic and molecular fingerprints of Alzheimer's patients linked to past medical practices. DNA examination of conserved samples, combined with developments in bioinformatics, allowed researchers to find commonalities and variations among affected individuals. This not only proved the transmission relationship but also provided insights into the mechanisms controlling the vulnerability of particular individuals to the transmitted disease.

The findings indicated a troubling sequence of repeated treatments with tainted growth hormone components over several years. It became obvious that the transmission was not a single incidence but rather a consequence of systemic flaws in the medical operations of that age. The research methodology, through its thorough reconstruction of events, permitted the production of a detailed timeline that underscored the gravity of the situation.

The significance of these results extends beyond understanding the historical spread of Alzheimer's disease. It serves as a sharp reminder of the significance of careful investigation of medical practices, even those thought advantageous at the time. The lessons acquired from this historical research have far-reaching consequences for modern healthcare procedures, underlining the need for robust safety controls and continual monitoring of medical interventions.

Decoding the past requires a deliberate effort, combining historical knowledge, medical skills, and technical developments. The research not only disclosed the transmission of Alzheimer's disease through obsolete growth hormone therapies but also highlighted the broader ramifications for healthcare practices. This journey into the past serves as a sobering reminder of the responsibility that comes with medical discoveries, imploring the current and future generations to prioritize patient safety and ethical issues in the quest for scientific development.

Insights from Medical Records and Case Studies

Exploring the historical spread of Alzheimer's disease through outmoded growth hormone therapy needs a detailed dive into medical data and case studies. These remarkable resources provide essential insights into the patterns, repercussions, and unanticipated implications of the procedures undertaken decades ago.

Unraveling the Medical Records

1. Archival Challenges and Triumphs

Navigating through decades-old medical records has inherent obstacles, from fading ink to outmoded record-keeping systems. However, diligent efforts by academics have found a plethora of evidence that sheds light on the prevalence and frequency of growth hormone therapy throughout the designated period.

2. Patient Profiles and Treatment History

Examining individual patient data is crucial to understanding the course of Alzheimer's transmission. Analyzing treatment histories uncovers a narrative of repeated exposures to tainted growth hormone, typically spanning several years. The association between the duration of treatment and the onset of Alzheimer's symptoms emerges as a crucial feature of the inquiry.

Insights from Case Studies

3. Identifying Transmission Mechanisms

Case studies serve a vital role in establishing how Alzheimer's disease is disseminated through medical procedures. By examining the experiences of individuals who experienced these therapies, researchers can uncover precise transmission mechanisms. This includes the mechanisms via which the contamination occurred and the diversity in susceptibility among patients.

4. Patterns and Anomalies

The evaluation of several case studies allows for the detection of trends and anomalies. Are there commonalities in the age of onset, symptom progression, or other factors among persons affected? Understanding these patterns can lead to a more detailed picture of how the disease manifested as a result of past medical practices.

5. Geographical Variances

Case studies also offer the possibility to examine geographical differences in the transmission of Alzheimer's. Were different places more significantly affected due to extensive usage of hazardous products or unique medical practices? Investigating these differences provides a full understanding of the scope and impact of historical transmission.

Methodological Rigor and Challenges

6. Rigor in Research Design

Rigorous research procedures are vital to establishing the legitimacy of findings. From selecting representative case studies to utilizing statistical analysis, researchers must ensure that their techniques stand up to examination. This requires collaboration with experts in neurology, epidemiology, and related domains to validate and strengthen the research framework.

7. Ethical Considerations in Case Study Analysis

Ethical issues are crucial when delving into personal medical histories. Ensuring confidentiality, gaining informed permission where possible, and presenting findings responsibly are ethical imperatives. The ethical issues encountered in analyzing cases from decades ago show the significance of applying present ethical principles to historical research.

Unveiling Patterns and Correlations

8. Connecting the Dots:

Growth Hormone Treatments and Alzheimer's Onset

Through a comprehensive review of medical data and case studies, researchers make correlations between growth hormone therapies and the future onset of Alzheimer's. Correlations may include dosage-related effects, cumulative exposure, and the involvement of individual genetic variables in amplifying vulnerability.

9.Long-term Consequences of Repeated Exposure

The investigation of case studies indicates the long-term repercussions of repeated exposure to polluted materials. This extends beyond the acute transmission of Alzheimer's to issues of overall health, lifespan, and the impact on affected persons and their families.

Bridging Past and Present

10. Informing Modern Healthcare Practices

The insights gathered from medical records and case studies bear substantial significance for modern healthcare procedures. They underline the significance of strong safety measures, regular monitoring, and the need for continued study to understand the potential long-term repercussions of medical procedures.

11. Guiding Future Research Endeavors

The knowledge obtained from previous case studies serves as a guiding beacon for future research endeavors. Identifying gaps in understanding, refining methodology, and investigating opportunities for preventive measures become essential components of the legacy of these insights.

In deciphering the secrets of Alzheimer's transmission through historical medical processes, insights from medical records and case studies stand as foundations of understanding. Each case tells a tale, giving a piece to the intricate puzzle of how outmoded growth hormone therapy unknowingly played a role in defining the trajectory of Alzheimer's disease. As we bridge the past and present, these insights not only reveal the effects of yesteryears but also pave the road for a safer and more informed future in healthcare.

Chapter 4

Implications for Today

Lessons Learned from Historical Medical Practices

The ramifications of uncovering the transmission of Alzheimer's disease through ancient medical practices are severe. As we delve into the lessons acquired from past practices, it becomes evident that understanding our medical history is vital for establishing a safer and more informed healthcare landscape today.

One of the key lessons is the significance of strong safety protocols in medical treatments. The usage of outmoded growth hormone treatments, tainted over several years, alludes to a breach of the norms of the past. Today, this revelation serves as a sharp reminder of the crucial necessity for strong quality control methods in the creation and administration of medical therapies. The advent of technology and enhanced regulatory frameworks allows us to execute more sophisticated safety checks, lowering the danger of unintended effects.

Moreover, the historical transmission of Alzheimer's disease highlights the necessity of extensive study and continual monitoring of medicinal interventions. As we evaluate the prior cases and trends, it becomes obvious that the long-term effects of certain therapies may not have been fully understood at the time of their administration. In the present, this underscores the requirement of continual research to completely review the safety and efficacy of medical operations, including those considered routine.

Ethical considerations frequently come to the forefront while thinking about earlier medical practices. The inadvertent transmission of Alzheimer's raises problems regarding informed consent, patient autonomy, and transparency in healthcare. Today, there is a heightened emphasis on respecting patients' rights and ensuring that they are fully informed about the potential risks and advantages of any medical intervention. The lessons learned from the past aid contemporary healthcare workers in sustaining ethical standards and creating trust between patients and practitioners.

Furthermore, the ramifications extend to public health policies and education. Understanding the historical transmission of Alzheimer's disease requires a reevaluation of how we teach both healthcare professionals and the general public about medical treatments. It emphasizes the necessity for clear communication, awareness initiatives, and comprehensive training to empower individuals with the knowledge to make educated decisions about their healthcare.

The revelation also supports a more proactive approach to preventative healthcare. By addressing the potential long-term repercussions of medical operations, healthcare organizations can prioritize preventative efforts and early diagnosis of disorders. This shift in focus coincides with the broader push towards individualized medicine and holistic healthcare, seeking not just to treat but also to prevent and reduce potential hazards.

In addition to these general teachings, there are specific implications for different medical specializations. Neurology, in particular, can benefit from a clearer understanding of the historical transmission of Alzheimer's. This insight may lead to more targeted research into the disease's roots and course, potentially uncovering new pathways for therapy and prevention.

The consequences for today from the historical transmission of Alzheimer's disease through medical treatments are varied. They ask for a reexamination of safety protocols, a commitment to ongoing research, a reinforcement of ethical norms, advances in public health education, and a proactive approach to preventative healthcare. By learning from the mistakes of the past, we can construct a more resilient and patient-centric healthcare system, better suited to tackle the difficulties of the present and future.

Contemporary Relevance and Healthcare Considerations

Contemporary Relevance and Healthcare Considerations

In the ever-evolving environment of healthcare, the recent revelation that Alzheimer's disease may have been spread through antiquated medical methods has spurred significant conversations on modern relevance and healthcare implications. This revelation not only gives insight into the historical backdrop but also promotes a reevaluation of contemporary practices to safeguard the well-being of patients. In this research, we look into the ramifications of these results on modern healthcare and the steps needed to negotiate the ethical and medical problems they provide.

Understanding the Historical Context

Before we address the modern ramifications, it's necessary to understand the historical backdrop of Alzheimer's disease spread through medical operations. The outmoded kind of growth hormone treatment, polluted over several years, has been identified as a potential vector for the spread of this devastating neurological condition. This historical insight serves as a sharp warning that medical treatments, even with the best intentions, can have unexpected consequences that endure for decades.

Lessons from the Past

One of the important issues for current healthcare is to draw valuable lessons from the past. The retrospective review of medical records and case studies from the era when these therapies were common helps us to detect trends and transmission pathways. This historical reflection provides a cornerstone for establishing methods to prevent similar oversights in modern medical procedures.

Ethical Dimensions of Modern Healthcare

The revelation of Alzheimer's transmission through medical procedures raises ethical problems that echo in today's healthcare scene. The role of healthcare providers to emphasize patient safety is paramount. This needs a reexamination of ethical principles and practices to guarantee that the benefits of medical interventions outweigh any hazards. As we confront the repercussions of previous oversights, it becomes vital to create a healthcare system that places patient well-being at its core.

Reevaluating Safety Protocols

In light of this historical revelation, current healthcare must examine and enhance safety protocols. Stringent procedures are essential to prevent the unintended transfer of illnesses through medical interventions. This requires not only evaluating the compounds used in therapies but also adopting thorough screening systems to identify potential dangers. Advancements in technology and diagnostic technologies can play a crucial role in increasing the safety net of healthcare systems.

Patient Awareness and Informed Consent

Empowering patients with knowledge about the risks and benefits of medical interventions is vital in the modern healthcare landscape. Informed consent takes on heightened relevance, and healthcare practitioners must participate in frank communication with patients. This guarantees that patients are actively involved in their healthcare decisions, understanding the potential risks connected with treatments and agreeing based on thorough information.

Collaborative Research for Prevention

The revelation of Alzheimer's transmission underlines the significance of coordinated research efforts to prevent future occurrences. The healthcare community, researchers, and legislators must collaborate to conduct comprehensive studies on the potential long-term implications of present medical practices. This collaborative approach can lead to the discovery of dangers, implementation of preventive measures, and ongoing improvement in healthcare protocols.

Shaping a Safer Medical Landscape

As we manage the present relevance of the Alzheimer's transmission finding, it is vital to cooperatively engage towards establishing a safer medical landscape. This entails continual education, continuous research, and the integration of developing technologies to enhance the precision and safety of medical operations. A proactive posture is vital in recognizing and addressing possible dangers before they become ubiquitous.

The finding of Alzheimer's transmission through obsolete medical techniques serves as a sobering reminder that healthcare is a dynamic area that demands continual observation and progress. Contemporary relevance and healthcare considerations need a proactive and collaborative approach to safeguard the safety and well-being of patients. By learning from the past, reevaluating ethical norms, reinforcing safety regulations, and fostering transparency, we can negotiate the intricacies of modern healthcare and strive for a future where unintended consequences are avoided, and patient safety remains paramount.

Chapter 5

Ethical Reflections

Examining the Ethical Dimensions of Past Practices

The news that Alzheimer's disease might have been transferred through obsolete growth hormone therapies raises fundamental ethical considerations regarding the medical practices of the past. In this section, we delve into the ethical reflections around these historical procedures, analyzing the ramifications for patients, healthcare providers, and society as a whole.

The Patient's Perspective

First and foremost, we must address the impact on persons who inadvertently had therapies that could have potentially transferred Alzheimer's disease. These patients placed their trust in medical personnel, expecting the best possible care. The ethical challenge comes as we ask whether these patients were provided with sufficient information about the hazards linked with the therapy. Informed consent is a cornerstone of ethical medical procedures, and the disclosure invites us to review whether this concept was respected during the era of these now obsolete growth hormone treatments.

Additionally, the long-term effects for persons suffering from Alzheimer's as a result of these surgeries cannot be overlooked. The ethical responsibility extends to addressing the well-being of these individuals, ensuring that sufficient support and resources are made available for their care and quality of life.

Healthcare Professional Accountability

Examining the ethical dimensions entails a critical review of the responsibilities of healthcare practitioners throughout the period in question. Were these practitioners aware of the potential dangers associated with the growth hormone therapy they administered? If so, did they explain these risks honestly to their patients? Assessing the ethical conduct of healthcare practitioners becomes critical in establishing if the principles of beneficence and non-maleficence were upheld.

This thought also extends to the medical community's response to increasing evidence and concerns. Did healthcare personnel actively engage in ethical conversations concerning the safety and efficacy of the treatments, or were there systemic obstacles that inhibited such discussions? Addressing these concerns helps us appreciate the ethical climate within the medical sector throughout the time of these surgeries.

Societal Impact and Trust in Healthcare

Beyond individual experiences, we must address the broader societal ramifications of knowing that a disease like Alzheimer's could have been mistakenly spread through medical procedures. The erosion of public trust in healthcare systems is a fundamental ethical concern. The disclosure raises questions about the transparency of medical institutions, their dedication to patient welfare, and the effectiveness of regulatory structures in place.

To recover and retain trust, it is vital that the healthcare business demonstrates accountability, openness, and a commitment to learning from past mistakes. Ethical considerations must govern attempts to improve communication between healthcare professionals and the public, ensuring that information about medical procedures and potential hazards is delivered in an accessible and intelligible manner.

Learning from the Past: Ethical Guidelines for Modern Healthcare

As we reflect on the ethical dimensions of historical practices, it provides a catalyst for building rigorous ethical principles in contemporary healthcare. Lessons acquired from the unintended transfer of Alzheimer's through outmoded treatments should inform contemporary procedures and policies. This entails a dedication to transparency, continual education, and a patient-centered approach to care.

Ensuring that ethical issues remain at the forefront of medical decision-making is vital for developing and maintaining trust in healthcare systems. This reflection on the past serves as a reminder of the ethical obligations that accompany developments in medical science and underscores the necessity for a continuing discourse regarding the ethical elements of healthcare practices.

In studying the ethical features of past practices connected to Alzheimer's therapy, we confront tough considerations concerning informed consent, healthcare professional accountability, society trust, and the lessons we must take forward. This reflection is not only an admission of previous failures but a call to action for the continuing advancement of ethical standards in healthcare. As we manage the intricacies of medical developments, our dedication to ethical considerations is vital, ensuring that the well-being of individuals and the trust of society is central to our healthcare practices.

Ensuring Patient Safety in Modern Healthcare

Patient safety is a crucial concern in contemporary healthcare, with the evolution of medical procedures and technology advancements. In light of findings of Alzheimer's disease transmission through obsolete growth hormone therapy, a thorough reconsideration of patient safety precautions becomes needed. This essay addresses the various facets of preserving patient safety in modern healthcare, analyzing lessons learned from historical errors and offering measures for a safer medical landscape.

The foundation of patient safety lies in a full understanding of potential dangers connected with medical interventions.

Learning from the historical background of Alzheimer's transmission, healthcare providers must analyze the safety of therapies, drugs, and procedures. Rigorous assessment and monitoring processes should be implemented to identify and reduce possible risks before they escalate. This proactive strategy guarantees that patients are shielded against unintended injury, consistent with the ethical duty to prioritize their well-being.

In the present day, technological innovations play a key role in promoting patient safety. Electronic health records (EHRs) promote smooth communication among healthcare practitioners, lowering the likelihood of errors due to misinterpretation or lack of information. Integrated systems allow real-time access to patient data, enabling teamwork and informed decision-making. Additionally, automated warnings and reminders inside these systems serve as protections, urging healthcare personnel to adhere to best practices and norms.

Standardization of protocols and processes is another key part of ensuring patient safety. Implementing evidence-based standards across healthcare facilities offers a standardized framework for diagnosis, treatment, and follow-up care. Standardized protocols not only enhance the quality of healthcare delivery but also eliminate deviations that might lead to errors. By developing a standard approach to patient care, healthcare institutions can limit the likelihood of adverse events and promote a culture of safety.

Education and training are the foundations of a safety-centric healthcare system. Healthcare personnel must undergo continual education to stay current with increasing medical knowledge, technological breakthroughs, and best practices. Training programs should emphasize not only professional abilities but also a thorough awareness of patient safety standards. Furthermore, promoting a culture of open communication and reporting within healthcare teams facilitates the detection and resolution of safety hazards at an early stage.

Transparency is a vital element in creating and sustaining confidence between healthcare practitioners and patients. Honest and open communication regarding potential hazards, treatment alternatives, and expected outcomes empowers patients to make informed decisions about their care. In circumstances where ambiguities exist, healthcare providers should freely communicate them with patients, supporting shared decision-making and building a collaborative approach to treatment.

In the field of pharmaceutical safety, severe safeguards must be in place to prevent errors in prescribing, dispensing, and administering medications. Barcoding technologies, electronic prescription, and drug reconciliation processes contribute to minimizing pharmaceutical-related errors. Regular audits and evaluations of medication practices, coupled with ongoing education for healthcare personnel, are critical components of a successful drug safety strategy.

Patient involvement is a vital component of a safety-centric healthcare system. Empowering people to actively participate in their care, ask questions, and communicate openly with healthcare providers develops a sense of collaboration. Patient feedback methods, including surveys and forums, provide significant insights into the effectiveness of safety measures and areas that require improvement.

Continuous quality improvement initiatives are crucial for maintaining and strengthening patient safety standards. Healthcare facilities should have rigorous procedures for monitoring, analyzing, and upgrading their safety protocols. Regular audits, incident reporting systems, and root cause analyses contribute to identifying systemic issues and executing corrective steps. By fostering a culture of continuous improvement, healthcare institutions demonstrate their dedication to providing safe and effective treatment.

In conclusion, protecting patient safety in modern healthcare demands a holistic and proactive strategy. By learning from historical lapses, embracing technology breakthroughs, standardizing processes, prioritizing education and training, promoting transparency, including patients, and cultivating a culture of continuous improvement, healthcare institutions may provide a safer environment for patients. As the healthcare landscape continues to evolve, the commitment to patient safety remains unbroken, reflecting the ethical obligation to prioritize the well-being of those entrusted to our care.

Chapter 6

Looking Forward

Future Research and Alzheimer's Prevention

The examination of future research and Alzheimer's prevention highlights a significant component of our path into understanding and resolving the effects of historical medical practices on the spread of this devastating disease. As we delve into this forward-looking perspective, it becomes obvious that the knowledge garnered from the revelations of past transmission cases should serve as a spark for proactive measures in the fields of research, prevention, and healthcare policy.

The key focus of future research rests in knowing the complicated mechanisms behind Alzheimer's transmission and progression. While past cases provide useful information, present scientific breakthroughs open options for more specific study. Researchers are progressively employing cutting-edge technology, such as enhanced imaging techniques and molecular analysis, to untangle the molecular and cellular subtleties linked with Alzheimer's disease. By examining the pathophysiological processes at a granular level, scientists attempt to uncover specific markers and targets that can be exploited for early identification and intervention.

One significant field of investigation is the role of genetics in Alzheimer's susceptibility and transmission. knowledge the interplay between hereditary characteristics and environmental effects, including past medical treatments, can provide a more detailed knowledge of individual predispositions. Genetic research provides the potential of personalized treatment, allowing for targeted interventions based on an individual's genetic profile, ultimately boosting the efficacy of prevention methods.

Moreover, the research of modifiable risk variables increases priority in the hunt for Alzheimer's prevention. Lifestyle decisions, such as food, exercise, and cognitive involvement, have been implicated in determining the risk of getting Alzheimer's disease. Future research attempts should delve deeper into these parameters, revealing the particular pathways via which they effect brain health. This understanding can be converted into targeted therapies and public health campaigns, encouraging individuals to choose lifestyle choices that promote cognitive well-being and minimize the risk of Alzheimer's.

Advancements in neuroimaging technologies also give a glimpse into the dynamic changes occurring in the brain during the preclinical stages of Alzheimer's. Longitudinal studies tracking individuals over time provide valuable data on the evolution of biomarkers associated with the disease. This not only aids in early diagnosis but also facilitates the identification of important moments for intervention. Early identification is crucial, as therapies undertaken during the preclinical phase hold more potential for slowing or preventing the progression of Alzheimer's.

The idea of preventive medicines and vaccinations is another area in Alzheimer's research. Building on the insights learnt from historical transmission cases, researchers are actively pursuing therapeutic techniques to minimize the chance of developing the condition. Vaccine development, in particular, bears promise in preparing the immune system to recognize and destroy pathogenic proteins linked in Alzheimer's, thereby preventing their accumulation in the brain.

Collaboration and interdisciplinary research are crucial in expanding our understanding of Alzheimer's and establishing effective preventive measures. The convergence of expertise from neurology, genetics, immunology, and other related domains supports a holistic approach to confronting the multiple character of the disease. Initiatives that stimulate cross-disciplinary collaboration and data-sharing are vital for expediting progress in Alzheimer's research.

Beyond the laboratory, the translation of research findings into meaningful policies is crucial. Healthcare systems must change to accommodate the growing landscape of Alzheimer's prevention. This involves incorporating risk assessments, genetic testing, and cognitive exams into standard healthcare processes. Public awareness campaigns can play a vital role in sharing knowledge about preventive measures, helping individuals to make educated decisions regarding their cognitive health.

The voyage of exposing Alzheimer's secrets continues beyond the historical setting into a future influenced by rigorous research, proactive prevention techniques, and ethical considerations. By utilizing improvements in technology, genetics, and preventative medicine, we are on the edge of transformational innovations that have the potential to alter our approach to Alzheimer's disease. The lessons learnt from the past move us toward a future where the transmission of Alzheimer's becomes an avoidable chapter in the annals of medical history.

Shaping a Safer Medical Landscape

In the wake of findings regarding the unintended transmission of Alzheimer's disease through obsolete growth hormone therapy, there is an urgent call to action for defining a safer medical landscape. The ramifications of ancient medical practices have cast a shadow on the healthcare profession, requiring a reevaluation of protocols and a commitment to ensure the safety of patients in the present period.

The route to designing a safer medical landscape begins with a careful review of the lessons acquired from the past. The use of now-obsolete growth hormone treatments, frequently provided repeatedly using contaminated material, serves as a sharp reminder of the unforeseen consequences that can come from antiquated medical methods. Understanding the core causes and transmission pathways is vital in averting such oversights in contemporary healthcare.

Modern medicine is at the convergence of technology breakthroughs and ethical considerations. As we negotiate this complex landscape, it is vital to integrate the knowledge learned from previous examples into present medical procedures. The adoption of rigorous screening systems, severe quality control measures, and ongoing monitoring can act as bulwarks against the recurrence of accidental disease transmissions.

One of the key obstacles is in striking a balance between medical innovation and patient safety. The hunt for cutting-edge treatments should be complemented by a solid system that prioritizes thorough testing, rigorous validation, and continual observation. Collaborations between medical researchers, practitioners, and regulatory organizations become important in developing and preserving these standards.

In the goal of a safer medical landscape, openness becomes a cornerstone. Open communication channels between healthcare professionals, researchers, and the public encourage trust and accountability. Patients have the right to be informed about the potential dangers involved with medical procedures, enabling them to make educated decisions regarding their health.

Education emerges as a crucial instrument in establishing a safer medical ecosystem. Healthcare practitioners must stay current of the newest research findings, evolving technologies, and best practices. Continuous training programs and knowledge-sharing activities can strengthen the competency of medical practitioners, equipping them to manage the dynamic healthcare environment with alertness and precision.

Ethical reflections on previous activities assist the formation of ethical rules for the future. The consideration of the ethical elements surrounding previous medical treatments employing tainted material invites a reevaluation of the principles that should govern medical research and treatment. Striking a balance between increasing medical knowledge and maintaining the well-being of patients is a delicate but vital task.

The integration of technological solutions also plays a crucial role in building a safer medical landscape. Advancements in diagnostic equipment, sterilizing processes, and treatment regimens contribute to decreasing the dangers involved with medical treatments. Embracing innovation while retaining a persistent commitment to patient safety symbolizes a harmonious convergence of development and responsibility.

As we move forward, the focus on prevention becomes paramount. Investing in research committed to understanding the potential long-term repercussions of medical procedures is crucial. Proactive approaches, such as detailed risk assessments and preventive initiatives, can assist mitigate unforeseen problems, ensuring that the medical environment remains a sanctuary for healing rather than a source of unintentional harm.

In conclusion, the imperative of "Shaping a Safer Medical Landscape" needs a holistic approach. Learning from the past, embracing transparency, promoting education, respecting ethical standards, integrating technology responsibly, and emphasizing prevention collectively constitute the blueprint for a healthcare system that promotes patient safety above everything. It is a shared obligation that transcends individual positions, requiring the collaborative commitment of healthcare professionals, researchers, politicians, and the public to establish an atmosphere where medical advancement coexists happily with unflinching patient safety.

Conclusion

Throughout our research into the historical spread of Alzheimer's disease through obsolete medical methods, we've embarked on a trip loaded with revelations, insights, and ethical dilemmas. The unraveling of this silent legacy sheds light not only on the past but also on the present and future of healthcare practices.

Our journey began with an awareness of the perplexing character of Alzheimer's dementia, an illness that has long confused researchers and clinicians alike. Despite decades of investigation, many riddles concerning its genesis and course remain unexplained. However, our inquiry into previous medical practices has found a crucial piece of the jigsaw, offering valuable background to understand the disease's transmission patterns.

In going into the historical context, we traced the origins of this revelation to the widespread usage of growth hormone treatments in the past. These medications, formerly touted as medical breakthroughs, were provided without full awareness of the potential consequences they posed. Repeated exposure to tainted material during these procedures inadvertently facilitated the transmission of Alzheimer's disease, setting the groundwork for a stealthy spread that would only be detected years later.

The process of exposing this buried history requires diligent research techniques and careful review of medical data and case studies. Through laborious study, patterns of transmission began to emerge, creating a picture of unknowing individuals who had unwittingly become victims of obsolete medical procedures. Each story provided as a sobering reminder of the significant influence that historical decisions may have on the health and well-being of individuals and communities.

As we ponder on the relevance of these discoveries for current healthcare, several crucial lessons come to the fore. Firstly, we are reminded of the significance of alertness in the face of medical progress. While breakthroughs in medicine hold the potential to improve health outcomes, they must be supported by rigorous oversight and examination to ensure patient safety. Secondly, the disclosure of Alzheimer's transmission through medical procedures underlines the interconnectivity of healthcare practices across time. What transpired decades ago continues to echo in the present, prompting us to address the legacy of past actions with humility and resolve.

Moreover, our investigation into this area involves ethical questions that deserve serious attention. How can we reconcile the desire for medical progress with the imperative to not harm? What obligations do healthcare practitioners and policymakers share in ensuring the well-being of patients both today and in the future? These are complicated topics that demand continual conversation and thought within the medical community and society at large.

Looking forward, our voyage finishes with a sense of cautious optimism tempered by a sober understanding of the challenges that lay ahead. While the revelation of Alzheimer's transmission through medical procedures constitutes an important milestone in our understanding of the illness, more work remains to be done. Continued study into its genesis, prevention, and treatment is necessary to lessen its impact on individuals and families globally.

In closing, the path of exposing Alzheimer's mysteries serves as a sad reminder of the ability of historical inquiry to enlighten and improve our approach to healthcare. By addressing the shadows of the past, we highlight pathways toward a healthier and more equitable future for all. Let us carry forward the lessons acquired from this trip with humility, empathy, and a steadfast commitment to the well-being of the people we serve.

www.ingramcontent.com/pod-product-compliance
Lightning Source LLC
Chambersburg PA
CBHW050042260726
48658CB00005B/1738